Pocket 1

Reiki

Chantal Dupont

Astrolog Publishing House

Pocket Healing Books

Holistic Healing
Dr. Ilona Melman

Aromatherapy
Kevin Hudson

Reiki
Chantal Dupont

Vitamins
Jon Tillman

What is Reiki?

The Japanese word *Reiki* consists of two words: *rei*, meaning "universal energy," and *ki*, meaning "life energy," which links the body, mind, and spirit. Reiki originated in the Far East - in Japan - where it was discovered, but it is an ancient energy whose power is similar to the marvelous healing powers of the ancient masters. It is transmitted personally from teacher to pupil. Reiki treatment is done by placing the hands on the body, and transmitting energy from the practitioner to the recipient. The practitioner (who can also treat himself!) serves as a channel for the universal healing energy that passes through him to the recipient.

Reiki was discovered by the Japanese theologian, Dr. Mikao Usui, at the end of the nineteenth century. Dr. Usui discovered the ancient healing art, which had been long forgotten by the world. He spent a great deal of time searching intensively for this ancient art, and performing an in-depth investigation of ancient laws of Buddha. After visiting a Zen monastery, Dr. Usui fasted and mortified his flesh on Mt. Kurama for a period of 21 days, during which he practiced asceticism and meditation. It was during this period, when Dr. Usui was granted enlightenment, that the path leading to the forces of universal healing opened up before him, and granted him the power of Reiki. This gift enabled Dr. Usui to transmit Reiki energy to others, and he taught them how to become a channel for this energy. In this way, the first great Reiki Masters received their training, among them Dr. Chujiro Hayashi, Hawayo Takato. and Phyllis Lei Furumoto. With the help of these great Masters, the art of Reiki reached the West, via personal training (attunement) and the training of additional teachers.

Reiki stimulates the life energy inside us. Reiki cannot be "imposed," nor can "too much" Reiki energy be transmitted to anyone, because the marvelous thing about Reiki energy is that it reaches the recipient in exactly the amount and manner that he is prepared to receive. In the same way, the power of Reiki healing is manifested. The more a person opens himself up to the wonderful energy, the greater the changes that will occur in his life. Of course, when we receive the gift of Reiki by means of training with a Master, the changes that are likely to occur in our lives are far-reaching.

Most of the problems that beset a person, as well as his motives in this world, are the result of "separation." Separation begins between the person and himself, and at the same time, between him and his God. When a person is not at one with himself, he is unable to feel the sensation of marvelous oneness with other people, and then it is possible to see all the regrettable manifestations of separation. People ask themselves, "Who am I really?", and have difficulty expressing - sometimes even acknowledging - their true feelings, sensations, motives, and desires. They vacillate between wishes and hidden passions on the one hand, and self-criticism and guilt feelings on the other, find it difficult to accept themselves, and for this reason, have a hard time accepting those around them, and what is happening in their world.

The feeling of oneness, which a person who has undergone Reiki training is likely to experience, is stunning in its power, and in its ability to change all one's patterns of life and thought, opening a new path to self-knowledge. Sometimes, during Reiki treatment, the practitioner and the recipient feel that they are one. The energy that flows between them unites them. This feeling of oneness is unique and extraordinary, and will probably cause the person to ask himself many existential questions that he was previously afraid to ask, repressing and concealing them instead.

When receiving Reiki, many physical and mental blockages may appear and be released. People will probably remember things and see scenes from their past, which provide certain answers pertaining to difficulties and hardships in the present. They may feel "strange" sensations, a sudden emotional openness sometimes, and even a flood of emotions that had been repressed for so long. But there is no need to worry. As we mentioned before, the recipient allows the energy to reach only the places whose release he can endure. Reiki cannot harm. The burst of emotion that he may experience is exactly what he wished for, and what he needed at that particular period of his life. Although the first encounter may be a little bit "alarming," there is never any danger in it.

The History of Reiki

The wonderful story of Reiki begins in mid-nineteenth century Japan. It is a story that transcends continents, religions, and races, and its origins reside in the obstinate search for the special healing treatment by touch, which is hinted at in ancient writings. At the time, Dr. Mikao Usui was the dean of a small Christian university in Kyoto. That period was a period of change in Japanese life, which began to be exposed to western culture. The innovations of the Industrial Revolution in the West rapidly began to make their mark in Japan. Dr. Mikao Usui was intimately acquainted with one aspect of western culture: Christianity.

His belief in the Bible and the holy scriptures was so

profound that while teaching his students the Bible and the New Testament, they asked him if he accepted the holy scriptures in letter and spirit. "Of course," he answered, continuing to read the healing miracles wrought by Jesus with his students. "If that is the case," his students went on, "where is that hidden power by means of which Jesus and his disciples performed far-reaching medical miracles? Where is that power?" Since Dr. Usui could not provide a satisfactory answer to his students' questions, he felt that it was his personal obligation to set out on a quest for the answers. The very day he was asked the questions, he resigned from his post, and went off in search of the answers to the astonishing questions.

Initially, Dr. Usui went to the United States, because most of his teachers were American missionaries. He thought that perhaps by a meticulous scrutiny of the Christian scriptures, he would discover the answers. However, he did not find any answers there either. When it occurred to him that Buddha, too, had far-reaching medical abilities, he decided to return to Japan, where he would try and find the answers to his questions: What are the marvelous divine healing powers described in the scriptures and in the stories about Buddha, and how is it possible to link up to them, to bring them back into this world, for the benefit of the suffering and the oppressed?

Dr. Usui commenced a thorough search among the Buddhist monasteries in Japan. He searched in the ancient Buddhist sutras, asked the abbots and monks in the monasteries, but always, whenever he requested information, material or any kind of clues about Buddha's ways of healing the body, he received the same answer: over time, healing work had become focused on the spirit only, and no documentation concerning

Buddha's marvelous methods of treating and healing the body was to be found. This answer tormented Dr. Usui. In the New Testament, as well as in the Bible, cases of healing the suffering body itself were described. The same was true in the many stories about Buddha. Where were all those ancient methods? How could they be accessed? And so Dr. Usui continued his search.

Although he had plenty of reasons to give up after trying so many different places, and after asking so many wise abbots and not receiving any answers, his spirit did not break. He continued searching until he reached an isolated Zen monastery, from which he received a little bit of encouragement. The venerable abbot was not surprised at Dr. Usui's questions. He agreed with him. Buddha had indeed been gifted with the ability to heal people's bodies. The fascinating question also piqued the old abbot, who suggested that Dr. Usui stay in the monastery, and continue his marvelous quest there, by reading the sutras and the ancient Japanese texts. His support heartened Dr. Usui, and strengthened his spirit; his courage was bolstered. However, even in the ancient Japanese texts, he was unable to find the answers to his questions.

He began to search in the ancient Chinese sutras, and by dint of the tremendous power of learning and research with which he was blessed, rapidly covered a substantial part of the contents of the ancient sutras that he managed to lay his hands on. Even in these sutras, however, Dr. Usui succeeded in finding very little information. He still refused to give up. Now he hoped to find the answer in the ancient Tibetan sutras. To that end, he had to learn Sanskrit, the ancient language in which the Tibetan sutras were written.

It seems that during the time that Dr. Usui went on his wonderful journey to northern India, to the

Himalayas, he was informed of the discovery of ancient scrolls containing extremely valuable information. We do not know if Dr. Usui actually got hold of those scrolls, but after the journey and after learning the Tibetan lotus sutras, Dr. Usui felt that he had the information, the intellectual answer, to his questions. This was not enough, of course. In order to heal with the help of these marvelous powers, he needed the inspiration of a superior force, a divine blessing.

Armed with his new knowledge, Dr. Usui returned to his friend, the abbot, with a new question: How is it possible to receive these powers and use them for the benefit of mankind? The two friends meditated together for a long time, in an attempt to receive an answer to the question. Finally, they realized that the only way was for Dr. Usui to undertake a journey to the holy mountain, Mt. Kurama, in the vicinity of Kyoto, where he would undertake a regime of fasting and meditation for 21 days.

Dr. Usui climbed the mountain. He reached a certain point, which faced east, and there he arranged a formation of 21 stones, each one indicating a day of fasting and meditation. By the time he reached the 21st stone, nothing special or extraordinary had happened yet. It was the time of the new moon, and the mountain was virtually in darkness. Dr. Usui prayed with all his heart for a divine answer. Suddenly, the dark sky was pierced by an unexpected trail of light. The strange light approached Dr. Usui rapidly, becoming larger as it came nearer. Dr. Usui began to feel afraid. He was seized by a powerful urge to get up and flee from that strange light, which was approaching and growing so quickly. However, deep inside him, he knew. That was it. That was no doubt the sign he had been awaiting for so long. He knew that, after so much searching, and for so long, he could not give in now. With a prodigious mental effort, he forced himself to stay put, come what may.

At the very instant his heart made the decision, the tremendous light reached him and struck him hard in the middle of the forehead. Dr. Usui thought that he had died. Millions of bubbles in every color of the rainbow danced in front of his eyes, and then suddenly changed into bubbles of shining white light, each bubble containing a three-dimensional Sanskrit character, drawn in gold. One after the other they appeared in front of his eyes, for just enough time for him to internalize them and engrave them in his memory.

When he felt that the wonderful inspiration of the force had been completed, Dr. Usui was filled with gratitude and joy. He opened his eyes. To his surprise, the sun was already high in the heavens, and a new day of light stretched out before him. Very excited, eager, and happy, he began to run down the mountain slopes. To his great surprise, after 21 days of fasting and endless walking, he felt so strong, so full of life! That was a miracle in itself. He ran, filled with enthusiasm, anticipating how he would tell his friend, the abbot, about the incredible process he had undergone. In his haste, he suddenly bumped into a stone, and stubbed his toe badly. Instinctively, in a wave of pain, he stooped to grasp his toe. To his tremendous surprise, a few seconds later, the bleeding stopped, and the pain ceased entirely! His toe had healed completely, in a few seconds.

Dr. Usui continued on his way. He reached a roadside inn, and went in for breakfast. The innkeeper noticed his monk's vestments, and understood from the appearance of his face and body that the man opposite him had just undergone a long and difficult fast. He begged him not to eat a full breakfast, and suggested special food, lean and suitable for consumption after such a long fast. It is

well known that overeating after a long fast is extremely
dangerous. But Dr. Usui did not heed the innkeeper's
pleas. He ate his breakfast to the last crumb, and to the
innkeeper's amazement, nothing untoward happened to
him!

Dr. Usui looked at the innkeeper's granddaughter,
who had served him his breakfast. Her jaw was swollen;
she had been suffering from terrible toothache for several
days. Her grandfather, the innkeeper, was too poor to
take her to a dentist in Kyoto, so when Dr. Usui offered
to try and heal the girl, he was overcome with gratitude
and filled with hope. Dr. Usui placed his hands on the
sides of the girl's face. Within a short time, the pain
began to recede, and the swelling went down
considerably, much to the surprise of the onlookers.

That was not the end of the miracles for the day,
however. When Dr. Usui reached the Zen monastery, he
found his friend, the abbot, suffering from the pain of a
severe attack of rheumatism. While he was telling the
abbot about the wonders he had seen on his journey, and
about the extraordinary things he had experienced, he
placed his hands on the painful areas of the abbot's
body. The pain diminished, became progressively
weaker, and finally ceased altogether. The abbot was
dumbfounded. The energetic man who had followed his
heart and his spirit, in a search for the wondrous healing
powers of Buddha and Jesus, had indeed found the
answer.

Now Dr. Usui asked the wise old abbot for his advice
about what to do with the wonderful healing powers he
had been granted. Again, the abbot encouraged him to
meditate in order to receive the answer. After a period of
meditation, contemplation, and discussion, he reached
the conclusion that he should go out and work with his
new-found powers in the beggars' quarter of Kyoto, in
the hopes of helping and treating the beggars so that

they could receive a new name, as was the custom, become "regular" people again, and integrate into society.

As soon as he arrived in the beggars' quarter, Dr. Usui got down to work. He treated and healed young and old, men, women and children among the wretched beggars. The results were fantastic. Many of the beggars, who were suffering from a wide range of diseases as a result of their way of life, ghastly sanitary conditions, and various accidents, were cured of their ailments. Many of them were cured completely.

Dr. Usui continued his sacred mission for seven years. However, to his great amazement, he began to notice familiar faces. People who had been cured by him were coming back for help; they were sick with strange new diseases, and their lives had not been rehabilitated. One of the beggars, a young man, seemed especially familiar to Dr. Usui. During one of his visits, Dr. Usui said, "You look familiar to me. Haven't I seen you before?" "Of course!" answered the young man. "I am one of the first people who came to you. You cured me, I got a new name, I started a new life. I found work. I even got married. But to tell you the truth, all that involved too much responsibility. It was much easier and simpler to be a beggar..."

Dr. Usui soon discovered many similar cases. His despair was overwhelming. "Where did I go wrong?" he asked himself in agony. However, he soon understood that with all the will in the world, and his amazing healing abilities, he had not succeeded in teaching these people two crucially important things: responsibility and gratitude. Now he understood that healing the soul and the spirit were just as important as healing the body. By giving the beggars Reiki without asking anything in return, without healing their souls and spirits, he had simply nurtured the beggar inside them. Now he understood the importance of giving energy, and receiving energy in return for the giving. These people had to give something in return for the energy, for the healing they had received, and they had to take personal responsibility for the healing process they were undergoing. That is the reason why there must be a payment for Reiki: as a sign of taking personal responsibility for the treatment, and a sign of the genuine will to be healed and to rehabilitate oneself.

That is how Dr. Usui devised the five famous Reiki principles. He quit the beggars' quarter, and began to disseminate his theory all over Japan. At the same time, he began to understand with crystal clarity the meaning of the symbols he had received on the mountain, and began to use them in order to train people in the art of Reiki, so that they would accept personal responsibility for their self-healing process and for their physical, mental, and spiritual health. Now he started to instruct, attune and train additional teachers. Toward his death, Dr. Usui initiated one of his most loyal pupils, Dr. Chujiro Hayashi, and transferred the responsibility for continuing his path to him. Dr. Hayashi accepted the responsibility for transmitting and disseminating Reiki, and established the first Reiki clinic in Tokyo.

The next great Reiki teacher became acquainted with Reiki via her personal pain and suffering. In 1935, Hawayo Takata, a young Japanese-American woman, came into the clinic. She was suffering from a large number of organic disturbances, and displayed the symptoms of severe depression, as a result of the death of her husband several years previously, on her face. Her body was debilitated from grief. Mrs. Takata was about to undergo a high-risk operation in Japan. One night, she heard the voice of her deceased husband imploring her not to have the operation. After she explained to her doctor that she did not intend to undergo the operation, he realized that she was absolutely adamant, and could not be persuaded otherwise. He suggested that she go to the Reiki clinic, which Dr. Hayashi was managing at the time. Mrs. Takata took his advice, and began to undergo Reiki treatment. To her amazement, there was an enormous improvement in her condition - both physical and emotional - and she was eventually cured of her ailments, all the while regaining her strength and *joie de vivre*. She was astounded at Reiki's healing power. She did not require better proof than that of its marvelous power: her health was completely restored, and she had gotten out of the painful cycle of disease and severe depression following the death of her husband.

Until that time, Reiki had been considered the preserve of men only. However, a woman of Mrs. Takata's strength and determination would not let an obstacle like that prevent her from learning the healing profession that had saved her life. As we know, until now, Reiki had transcended continents, religions, and languages, and had been acquired as a result of a persistent search, without favoring one belief over any other. Now it would also become a symbol of the equality between the sexes, with Mrs. Takata receiving the first-degree attunement and training, followed soon after by the second-degree attunement and training. Mrs. Takata returned to the United States, bringing with her the new healing news.

Some time after she began her healing work in the United States, Dr. Hayashi and his daughter came to visit her. During the visit, Mrs. Takata was initiated as a "Reiki Master," and Dr. Hayashi and his daughter returned to Japan, secure in the knowledge that the work was being performed superbly by a faithful envoy in the

United States. As a result of his extraordinarily honed senses, Dr. Hayashi sensed, upon his return to Japan, the approaching war, which would create a deep chasm between Japan and the United States. With his sharp senses, he also understood what the consequences of this terrible war would be. Mrs. Takata, whose senses picked up his concern, went to Japan, where Dr. Hayashi told her of his fears. He felt that he had completed his mission here, and had decided to go on a long journey to the world beyond. In the presence of close friends, clothed in the appropriate ceremonial robes, Dr. Hayashi left his body in a conscious way. Mrs. Takata remained in Japan for some time in order to assist with the funeral arrangements, and from there went on to Hawaii in order to avoid the American-Japanese conflict of World War II.

After the war, Mrs. Takata returned to the United States, where she continued to disseminate Reiki, train many people, and heal many others. During the seventies, Mrs. Takata began to initiate other Reiki Masters. She passed away at the end of 1980, leaving many followers behind her. Since then, hundreds of Masters have been initiated, and thousands of other people have studied Reiki at various levels. The number of people whose lives have been transformed by Reiki, or whose physical health and mental and spiritual equilibrium have been restored by Reiki, is enormous. Dr. Mikao Usui's search for the path of marvelous healing was not futile. It lives and breathes to this very day, provides help, serenity, and health to hundreds of thousands of people worldwide.

Attunement: Receiving the Ability to Heal and to be a Reiki Channel

The Reiki pupil's ability to transmit Reiki can only be acquired from a Reiki Master. This unique way of receiving the ability to heal in a direct and energetic way from the Master differentiates Reiki from many other methods of holistic and energetic treatment.

In the attunement ceremony, which constitutes part of the Reiki course, the Master transmits the ability to be a channel for the universal Reiki energies to the pupil. For this reason, the ability to receive the healing powers of Reiki is so fast and permanent. From the moment a person has received the ability to be a Reiki channel, it will never abandon him. Even if he does not use his power for twenty years, when he eventually does want to transmit Reiki, he will find that he has not lost the power to do so. This is a lesson for the ego. We receive such an astounding power to heal without making any "effort," unlike other healing professions and other methods of healing by touch. We cannot take ego-boosting "credit" for ourselves, but we can just understand that those powers exist all the time, everywhere, and all we need to do is link up with them and let them perform the action of healing. Ultimately, we only serve as a channel for this healing energy, and when the energy passes through us, and when we transmit it to another person or creature, we ourselves are healed. From the moment the person receives the ability to heal from the Master, this ability will stay with him forever. It is possible that if he does not use it, it will diminish somewhat - so it would appear. But from the moment he resumes using it, the more regularly he uses it, the more it will strengthen and increase.

The Principles of Reiki

As we mentioned before, Reiki is likely to open up a new world of awareness and understanding to the student or recipient. The principles of Reiki help both the practitioner and the recipient absorb new insights, and cope with awareness in a better and clearer form. The principles serve as direction, points of light along the path, that direct the person gently to the appropriate place.

The first principle:
Just for today - I will not get angry.

Anger, irritation, nervousness. It's so easy to get angry. Sometimes, we do not look into the depths of the things that make us angry. We don't look into the depths of the feeling of anger. The smallest, dumbest things can get us into the bad and dangerous state of anger. Dangerous for us, and dangerous for others. How many times do we vent our anger on another person for some trifling reason, while the seed of the anger is planted somewhere deep in our beings, and is whipped out and explodes as a result of some minor, worthless trigger? The extent to which anger hurts us, first of all, and our surroundings, can be seen if only we open our eyes and look. So many people allow their ego, their fear of losing control, to rule their lives, to harm themselves and those around them, and to turn life into a long journey of power struggles, wars and angers. It sometimes seems as if anger is an infectious disease. It is rare to see smiling faces in the company of an angry person. Everyone is harmed by his wrath, to some extent, and some of them take on the anger that is thrown at them, and transmit it onward, hurting more and more people. People who allow their egos and their anger to direct their lives move farther and farther away from their "upper I," from their inner truth, which conceals itself in signs of anger. For how is it possible to be angry without completely ignoring our inner guide, the divine seed that is inside us, the pure truth? In order to be angry, to get irritated or to hurt others, we have to ignore them completely, not heed them, move as far away from them as possible. The farther we move away from the divine seed inside us, the more it seems that it is moving farther and farther away from us.

When we permit our ego to lead us, we suffer from futile expectations, desires, and wishes - sometimes to the point of being destructive. How many people have we seen getting angry and becoming enraged because of an injury to their honor or ego? How is it possible to live a harmonious and natural life when the ego and anger control that life? The non-realization of wishes that originate in our ego, and not in our inner truth or guidance, is liable to turn our lives into a series of endless disappointments, sorrow, and angers. What's more, when we learn to accept things as they are, when they cannot be changed, we gain peace of mind and serenity.

We often get angry because the people around us do not react in the way we want to our demands and expectations. But we have to remember: we are surrounded by people who in fact act as mirror images, or "inverted" mirror images, of us ourselves - "The pot calling the kettle black." It is amusing to see just how angry people can get about exactly those characteristics that they themselves have - instead of using the useful "mirror" that they elected to put up opposite them when they created those ties with the people around them. It would be funny, if it weren't so sad, to see how many parents get angry with their children, completely forgetting that they were the ones who served as an example and helped them become what they are now!

One of the most important spiritual studies is acknowledging that every situation we face is a kind of "lesson" that teaches us something. It is clear that when we react angrily, we do not learn the lesson, but rather repeat the same mistake over and over again.

When we look deeply into our personal lives, we can notice how much our beliefs and thoughts shape the reality in which we live. Thoughts of anger, fury, and resentment will ricochet at us like boomerangs, and then we will have to cope with the blow that we basically aimed at ourselves.

Is it possible to say, "I understand the meaning of anger, this non-positive and unwanted energy, and I will never get angry"? It is not easy to commit to that ... but if we remember this principle: Just for today - I will not get angry; I will not get irritable. What for? What's the use of those non-positive emotions? Will anger change anything? Will it repair whatever is broken, will it move the clock back, will it change the situation? No. It can only make things worse. If we remember, just for today, for this moment, right now, not to get angry; not to get irritable; to do what we have to do calmly, to change what can be changed, and to accept what can't - we will already have taken a significant step toward changing our entire way of life. Just for today - not to get angry, and not to get irritable.

> ## The second principle:
> ## Just for today - I will not worry.

Worry. Such a commonplace concept, so banal. But actually, when we know that our private providence is looking after us, when we have complete faith in ourselves and in God, is there room for worry? When we know that everything has a reason and a purpose in theuniverse, why must we worry?

Worry about the past, which takes up a lot of time and energy in many people's lives, is so unnecessary. We did the best we could in the situations we found ourselves in, according to the wisdom, the knowledge, and the awareness that we had at the time. We can learn lessons, learn, and become wiser, but why worry? Worry is such a passive emotion. It does not change things - not for the good, in any event. Worries about the past consume a lot of energy and forces that we need in order to get on with our lives here and now. Why torture ourselves with worries about the past? What's the use? Learning and drawing conclusions from the past are not worry, but rather a process of awareness and understanding, while resigning ourselves to what can no longer be changed, and changing what we are able to change - here and now.

Worry about the present is also superfluous and even dangerous. We create our future, and everything that comes to us is part of a plan of prodigious dimensions, in which we star like leading actors, and we have our personal power to change the course of things in the universal plan that has been prepared for us. Everything that happens to us has a reason and a purpose. Many things that happen are often things that we ourselves invited into our reality by means of our various worries and fears. Our worries and fears are also liable to realize themselves when we nourish them and invest energy and strength in them.

Why worry? If we remember, just for today, for the moment, here and now, not to worry, to do what we have to do calmly, to change what can be changed, and to accept what cannot be changed, we will already have taken a significant step toward changing our whole life. Just for today, I will not worry. When we stop worrying, will nothing work out as we wanted? Will our worry about money, the family, the car that has broken down, safeguard our family? Help us increase our monthly income? Repair the car? What is the use of worrying? The dangers in all those non-positive emotions are enormous. Physically, mentally, spiritually-energetically, and of course, environmentally. Many people tend to project their worries onto others, infect them with their fears and worries, or hold them back as a result of their irrational and illogical worries. Why should we spread our mental diseases and unbalanced states throughout the environment, infecting everything around us? Why must we introduce negative events into our emerging reality - out of worry for the people around us? Therefore, we have to remember: Just for today - not to worry; to live life as it is, without shouldering unnecessary and useless burdens.

The third principle: Just for today - I will earn a living honestly and decently, and I will do my work with integrity.

Honesty and decency do not have many faces - only one single truth, which we know inside ourselves. Nevertheless, internal manipulations are liable to condone things that are not honest or decent. People tend to say to themselves, "What could happen if I cut corners here or there? Nobody would know..." This attitude, however, is one of the sources of many evils in today's society. When a person adopts this approach, how can he believe in his fellow-man's honesty? How can he look at his own truth, or look himself in the eye?

The path to linking up with the "upper I," with self-recognition, passes through basic honesty and decency. Doing our work the best we can, honestly and decently, is one of the ways to link up with our inner truth. When work is done dishonestly, and not wholeheartedly, not out of truth and decency, we do not feel really worthy and deserving of recompense. Deep inside, we know that we did not do *perfectly* what we ourselves chose to take upon ourselves. How many frustrations, distresses, internal and external conflicts, and arguments with ourselves and with those around us could be avoided if we only did our work - and it makes no difference what kind of work - out of inner decency and honesty? This way is not only more pleasant - it is also easier and simpler.

When we talk about work, we do not only mean work for the sake of earning a living. We also mean inner work, work on ourselves. Here too, it is very easy to cut corners. But in order to enjoy a harmonious life -

both inner and outer - we have to do this work honestly and decently. The aim of this principle is to develop our inner honesty and decency so that they are manifested in every facet of our lives, and make our lives more serene, full, and pleasant When a person searches for his own truth, he has to search for the truth in everything, in his every deed. It is very easy to say, "Tomorrow I'll start acting honestly and decently in my inner work and my outer work, and with those around me." Not tomorrow, but now, in the present. Therefore, just for today, I will do my work honestly and decently.

The fourth principle:
Just for today - I will be grateful. (I will give thanks for the blessings in my life.)

Many people are outraged by this principle. What blessings? Many people are inclined to view their lives as a sequence of things that "have to be done," tasks, debts, difficulties that have to be coped with, sorrow, and tribulations. "What is there to be grateful about? What blessings?" they ask, completely forgetting the many tremendous blessings that they have in their lives. Of course, the first and foremost of them is the very fact that they are alive.

It is said that even in the most difficult situation, there are still rays of light to be grateful for. Many people enjoy good health, a family, friends, a roof over their heads, morning sunshine, birds chirping, without noticing that these things are wonderful, and they must rejoice and be thankful. Sometimes, their lives pass by without their being grateful for all the wonderful things in them.

When we live our lives acknowledging everything

we have been given and are lucky enough to have, and what we hope and believe that we will be given, we attract additional abundance, happiness, prosperity, and joy to ourselves. Life that is lived with gratitude becomes a life that is full of satisfying and joyous reasons to be grateful. Everything we focus on, and provide with the energy of thought and senses, increases. To the same extent, if we focus on lack, sadness, or the "have not" in our lives, those things will increase. And the opposite. When we live according to the principle of "Who is happy? The one who is satisfied with his lot," the lot that we are happy about, the "have" in our lives, upon which we focus and for which we are grateful, will increase. Focusing on lack, deprivation, all the while wanting and tending to live in the illusion that we are lacking, is one of the reasons for greed and avarice, which stem from that fear of lack. When we focus on what we have, on the wonderful blessings we are blessed with every moment and every day, not only will we increase the abundance of those blessings, but we will also live in a feeling of constant satisfaction and happiness.

> # The fifth principle: Just for today - I will show love and respect for every creature and every form of life

By forgetting this principle, forgetting the obvious fact that we - human beings, animals, plants, and nature - are all one and the same, a single living and inseparable tissue, we now live in a world filled with wars, smog, air pollution, a damaged ecological infrastructure that is constantly showing its bruised face through climatic changes and natural disasters, and a sharp drop in the standard of living and health of human beings, as a result of their merciless abuse of the environment. If people only observed this principle, so much sorrow and suffering in the world would be spared people and animals, not to mention the planet Earth, which is the victim of the urges of people who try with all their might to subjugate nature and control it, instead of living in harmony with it. Every attempt to imagine a world in which its creatures observe this golden principle broadens the heart and fills it with wonderful hopes for peace, brotherhood, and natural unity.

It is very easy to expect the other person to show us love and respect. Many people are inclined to say, "Let others first relate to us nicely, and welcome us, then we'll relate to them in the same way." However, we have to learn that every change begins with "I myself," always, and the first organism toward which we have to show love and respect is ourselves. The meaning of the sentence, "Love thy neighbor as thyself," embodies the open secret: only genuine self-love - and this does not mean the illusions of the ego, but rather healthy and normal self-esteem - will enable us to show that same esteem, respect, and love toward the rest of humanity and the living creatures that surround us.

The perception of the environment, animals, plants, and other people as different and separate from us is the root of the many ills that society suffered from in the past, and still suffers from now. When we understand that we are all dependent on the tight and inseparable connection on one another, and on our environment, we feel a natural and pleasant commitment to show our love and esteem to the world. This attitude grants us love and esteem from the world sevenfold. When we are aware that we are, at our source, energetic beings, as are all the different life forms around us, we understand that barriers of religion, race, sex, or form do not exist at all, but are just an illusion of our human perception, which we have to cope with. In fact, when we show our love and esteem toward every living creature and to every life form, we ultimately show love and esteem toward ourselves. The value of this principle is worth more than gold. When we use it on a daily basis to show and feel love and respect toward every living creature and every life form, we heal ourselves, those around us, and the world we live in.

The profound understanding of the Reiki principles, assimilating and remembering them in everyday life, will turn the Reiki that we receive or transmit into a way of life, while taking responsibility for our lives, health, and emotions.

How does Reiki work?

Our energy field, which also includes our physical body, is extremely sensitive to the energy of thought and the energy of feelings. When we experience within ourselves negative feelings or thoughts toward ourselves and the world, or develop negative thought patterns and non-positive and futile beliefs, this will soon be manifested in an overall influence on our energy field, on our feelings, on our health and on our entire way of life. When we experience these negative inner situations, the natural and normal energy flow in our bodies is disrupted, and various energetic, emotional, and physiological barriers occur and appear.

Reiki energy helps open these barriers, flows through all the blocked places, and moves the blocked energy, while cleansing blockages and helping the inner energy flow in a balanced, healthy, and correct way. Reiki energy penetrates all the blocked places - in the energetic bodies, and in the physical body. It strengthens the entire organism, reinforces the vital and life force, and strengthens the body's natural healing and regenerative power. Reiki energy strengthens the chakras and the meridians, so that life energy can pass more easily through our body and around our ethereal and energetic bodies.

In the case of various diseases, Reiki energy does not simply reinforce the body's natural power to fight disease, but it also opens up the mental layer to an understanding of why we "earned" those diseases, and what lesson they are teaching us. For that reason, there are sometimes cases wherein a person who is treated with Reiki first gains mental, spiritual, or emotional openness, but still feels no improvement in his physical condition. This is not coincidental in the least. Because Reiki energy is activated by the highest intelligence, it reaches the areas that need it - in the physical body, or in the various energetic bodies. To the same extent, it reaches the person in exactly the amount that he can receive, whether it is a lot or a little, and treats the layer that it is most important to open and balance immediately. Thus there are cases in which it seems that physical changes or relief cannot be seen immediately in the recipient's physical condition. In these cases, it seems that first and foremost, the other layers - mental, emotional, thought, and spiritual - must be worked on in order to enable the disease to be cured in such a manner that it will not recur in the same way, or in any other way, as a result of its mental, thought, or spiritual causes still not having been treated.

Many people suppose that various holistic or energetic treatments work as a result of the "power of belief," or various psychological effects. There is no doubt that this is not the case with Reiki. You do not have to believe in Reiki in order for it to work. It simply does what it has to do, whether you believe in it or not. To the same extent, it also influences animals and plants clearly and significantly, and it is impossible to claim that there is any kind of psychological effect on them, since they have no psychological awareness concerning the treatment they are being administered. However, they most certainly feel it, and sometimes even "ask" for it.

Having said that, it is extremely important for the person to want to be healed, in order to feel the obvious results of Reiki. In many cases, it is not possible to heal a person who does not want to let go of his disease. The desire to be healed is also manifested in the changes the person introduces into his way of life, his behavior patterns, his thinking and inner beliefs, which were almost certainly responsible for the onset of the disease or problem in the first place. Receiving, studying, or giving Reiki is sure to help the person cope with these changes in a better and more correct way.

Reiki's Influence on Our Quality of Life

One of the most dangerous enemies of a healthy, serene, and balanced life is stress, pressure, or tension. In the present fast-moving, materialistic, and achievement-oriented society, the daily pressures that people have to cope with are extremely heavy, and one can easily find oneself in situations of stress or tension at work, on the highway, at home - in fact, almost anywhere.

Stress or tension is a physical phenomenon to all intents and purposes. The emotional procedure that causes stress activates physical mechanisms. Finding oneself constantly in situations of pressure and tension exhausts the body as a result of the repeated and persistent activation of these mechanisms, which, from an evolutionary point of view, were meant to serve us in life-threatening situations of stress or tension, so as to make our attack or escape action more effective. Today, however, they are activated over and over again in many people during the course of the entire day. Situations such as falling behind schedule at work, family disputes, study pressures, and excessive demands from children, as well as a lack of consideration for their feelings or emotions, driving along the highway, financial pressures, and so on - all these cause tension, and gradually undermine all the body's systems.

Being in a constant state of stress is liable to

exhaust the person mentally and physically, and to expose and create various diseases. Reiki, administered regularly, exerts an enormous influence on reducing the stress from which modern man suffers so constantly. Lowering the level of stress is a continuous function of transmitting Reiki energy, and its major significance, besides the immediate sensation that is experienced when receiving Reiki, is the change in perception that frequently occurs in people who are treated with Reiki on a regular basis. Getting into a stressful state is a very subjective matter. Certain people are easily stressed out by things that appear "trivial" to others, while other people have a calmer and more serene - and therefore healthier - nature. The wonderful thing about Reiki is that it helps people get things into proportion, so that the pressure that is exerted on them becomes weaker as a result of their inner perception and the change in their view of life. Reducing stress and pressure helps the person in every aspect of life, strengthens him physically and mentally, and helps him maintain a healthy body and a stress-free mind.

Another area in which it is possible to see the influence of ongoing Reiki treatment is that of emotional balance. Similar to the situations of stress that we experience every day, there are also many emotional roller-coasters from which many people suffer constantly. Mood swings, ups and downs, feelings that are not harmonious, and many emotional states that persistently weigh on our nervous system, debilitate the immune system, harm the body as well as the thought and emotional layers, and sometimes cause people to get stuck on negative emotions and thoughts, as a result of which a gloomy, sad, and joyless picture of the world and of reality is created to a greater or lesser degree. It is wonderful to see how effective receiving

Reiki regularly is in helping to balance these emotional roller-coasters, and the way in which we interpret, accept, and work through various emotional states. States that would have previously inspired anger, sadness, an emotional outburst, sorrow or irritation in a particular person are now taken on board and interpreted in a far calmer and more relaxed manner after regular treatment with Reiki. And what happens when all those emotionally unbalanced states calm down? The enormous amount of energy that was invested in coping with those states, and with all those emotions that exhausted body and soul, now accumulates in marvelous "reserves" of energy that can be channeled along beneficial and useful paths.

Treatment with Reiki

The general action of Reiki on body and soul can be summed up in five main effects, which operate in tandem, and allow one another to work synergistically. First and foremost, as we mentioned previously, Reiki causes a sensation of profound calm. This factor is manifested strongly when practitioners in other fields of treatment by touch, such as massage or reflexology, who have undergone Reiki training, use these methods of treatment. Reiki is unlimited, and is transmitted during massage, Shiatsu, reflexology, and so on, while inducing a deeper state of calm in the recipient.

The profound calm and the feeling of release and relaxation bring about the second effect, which is the opening of energetic blockages. This effect may be manifested both in body and soul, and sometimes even invokes "forgotten" or repressed feelings, and helps the recipient understand them better.

The release of tension and pressure, and the opening of the physical and emotional blockages brings about the third effect of Reiki, which is the action of detoxifying the body. The release of the blockages affords a more harmonious, healthy, and balanced flow of life energy through the areas that had previously been blocked. In this way, Reiki helps balance and increase the body's action of draining and excreting the toxins that accumulate in the tissues, as well as the toxins that are not "physical," that is, the waste products of emotional and mental "pollution."

The fourth effect is the transmission of the universal healing energies, which reach the recipient in exactly the required quantity, and work on the layers that are in need of healing. After the body purifies itself of the various toxins in it, it has a greater capacity to receive the universal life force energy that comes to it via Reiki, and store it and use it.

This leads us to the fifth effect, which is raising and increasing the body's inner healing power - at the same time reinforcing the aura and increasing the person's vitality - when the universal healing power begins to exert its healing and curing action on it.

All these effects together cause the person to open up more to the cosmic forces, to become more spiritually refined, and broaden and deepen his spiritual ability, while regular Reiki treatments strengthen his body and soul, and enable him to feel physically and emotionally balanced.

Besides this general description of Reiki's action, it must be remembered that Reiki affects everyone differently and individually. The results of the Reiki treatment are actually determined by the needs of the recipient, which are not always obvious and conscious. Among the widespread results are emotional balance, which we spoke about before, release of blockages, including emotional ones, leading to emotional openness, release from stress, the balancing of energies that operate in the recipient's body, increased creativity, a feeling of replenished energy and physical energetic strengthening, increased awareness, and, of course, healing and relief from the diseases suffered by the recipient.

One of Reiki's most significant qualities, which makes it unique vis-a-vis many other holistic therapies, is the possibility of giving Reiki treatment any time, anywhere. It is possible to administer treatment in order to alleviate a particular pain, such as a headache or a stomach-ache, even in a crowded place such as a restaurant or a pub. Having said that, there are several important rules that should be strictly observed when we want to administer a complete or optimal treatment. It is best if the treatment is administered in a suitably aired room, without cigarette smoke or various chemical odors. The lighting should be low-key - preferably from a light that can be dimmed, or a candle; an essential oil burner with suitable aromatic oil can be placed in the room (it should be a genuine, pure oil, not a synthetic substitute); it is possible to play appropriately soft and gentle music, which will help the recipient enter a state of calm and serenity, or will distract him from disturbing thoughts. It is worthwhile checking that the music is compatible with the recipient, as well as the odor of the essential oil, since there are people who are bothered by these things for various reasons. It is important to choose a soothing oil such as lavender, frankincense, jasmine, and so on.

During the treatment, which can be performed when the recipient is either sitting or lying down, or even standing up, using techniques that will be described below, you must ensure that the recipient is in a comfortable position. If he needs a pillow while lying down, he should be given a comfortable pillow; sometimes a pillow under the legs is necessary for people who have an abnormally deep curve of the spinal column (lordosis). An extremely important factor to take note of is that the recipient must under no circumstances cross his arms or legs, so as not to cause blockages in the flow of energy. For that matter, the practitioner must also ensure that he himself does not cross his arms or his legs, or have one leg resting on the other.

As we said before, Reiki can be given in places where it is seemingly impossible to administer treatment, such as crowded places, or on a bus or a train, but the rule of not crossing arms or legs is possible and important to apply everywhere.

Reiki treatment is administered from the top down. When we give a "quick treatment" in order to relieve some kind of pain, we observe this rule, but we can concentrate just or mainly on the painful areas, or on the places in which we see a particular imbalance.

How to Place the Hands

During Reiki treatment, the palms must be turned downward, with the fingers close together and slightly curved. When we place our hands on our body, or on the recipient's body, we do not press hard, but rather just place our hands gently. Both hands are placed simultaneously on the area that is being treated, making sure not to cross them. When it is a place that is one of a pair, like the shoulders, we place one hand on each shoulder. It is also possible to place the hands one after the other, if necessary or convenient, but not one on top of the other. When we want to place our hand on a sensitive area such as the groin, we do not physically place our hand on the region, because of its great sensitivity, but we hold our hand five to seven centimeters above it.

In general, it is possible to perform a touch-free Reiki treatment simply by holding our hands at a distance of five to seven centimeters above the body, and treating it in the regular way. For this reason, even people who shy away from any kind of contact with the opposite sex, for religious or other reasons, can undergo or administer Reiki treatments with impunity, since it is possible to perform the treatment without physical contact.

When administering Reiki, there is an important point to remember. In principle, we do not "let go" or break contact with the recipient's body when moving from one hand location to the next. It is very important to ensure constant contact. When we want to descend from one point to the next, we first move one hand to the next point, while the other hand is still on the previous point, and then we move the other. When we ask the recipient to turn over from his back to his stomach and so on, we should leave one or both hands placed gently on a specific point on his body even while he is turning over, in order not to break contact. If for some reason it is not possible to leave our hand on the recipient's body when he changes his position, it is important to "imagine" that we are leaving our hand on his body or on the region of his aura. The same applies, of course, to a treatment in which for some reason or other, the practitioner may not place his hands on the recipient's body.

At the conclusion of the treatment, we do not

remove our hands from the recipient's body in a sudden, sharp movement, but rather very slowly and gently. There are Reiki Masters who teach various concluding movements. One of them, which is very widespread, is similar to the "time out" movement in basketball, and its aim is to announce, from the energetic point of view, that the treatment has been completed.

Self-Treatment with Reiki

Many Masters not only encourage their pupils to try self-treatment with Reiki, but actually insist that they do so. And rightfully. In fact, this is one of the most powerful ways to understand Reiki's tremendous contribution to every aspect of life, and even more than that, to begin to understand intuitively and via feelings what Reiki really is. In order to illustrate this point, we present the story of Jesse, today a Reiki master who runs workshops for teaching Reiki.

Jesse, 45 years old, lived an ostensibly ordinary life, without getting too involved in "the meaning of life," as he would put it, using a slightly derogatory tone that reflected his attitude toward the various theories pertaining to self-awareness, universal energies, and so on. He was a successful businessman, married, and father of two grown children, and he lived his life according to patterns he had acquired throughout his life - some of them inhibiting and treacherous, of which he was unaware. His life flowed more or less smoothly, until the accident. When he was 40, Jesse was badly injured in a serious automobile accident. He was hospitalized for a long time with a serious spinal injury as well as a head injury that caused him speech and other functional problems. The accident destroyed his world in the blink of an eye. From a strong, authoritative man who was confident that he was in absolute control of his life, he suddenly became a helpless person who was going through a difficult period of recuperation.

That wasn't the end of his troubles, however. While he expected full support from his immediate family, it transpired that his wife was unable - and perhaps even unwilling - to deal with the serious repercussions of the accident on their lives. While Jesse was a successful businessman, a strong, impressive man, she stood at his side. Now that he was unable to return to work, both because the physical and verbal injury, and because of the mental trauma he was forced to cope with, serious cracks began to appear in the couple's relationship. Broken-hearted, Jesse realized that he had given his heart to a women who was unable to stand by him in times of trouble. The sticky divorce added considerably to his difficulties in coping with and adapting to his new situation, and the need to virtually start a new life because of his physical limitations.

As a strong and determined man, Jesse succeeded in overcoming, to some extent, most of the difficulties. His physical rehabilitation was quite good, but the scars - both physical and mental - left their mark on him. He became a bitter person, lacking in confidence in life and in the order of the universe, which had been so cruel to him, and restless, intolerant and irascible in the extreme. These traits, of course, made his life even harder, and although he had recovered quite well from the physical point of view, he had a hard time finding a mate and leading a satisfying and enjoyable life.

In addition to the difficulties in finding work in his present state, Jesse suffered from extremely severe back pains that were so powerful that they sometimes neutralized him. He tried all kinds of treatments, from physiotherapy to various surgical procedures. But nothing helped. Ultimately, his physicians gave him to understand that the pains would be a part of his life forever. Jesse was not prepared to accept this, however. While he was suffering from such agonizing pain, his chances of rebuilding his life fully and well, of working in a satisfying job where he could realize his talents, and even of "calming down" a bit, seemed infinitesimal. He refused to resign himself to the facts.

During a sojourn in a special clinic for people who suffered from chronic problems and severe pain, Jesse met a Reiki practitioner. She was a friendly and tolerant person, and managed to see beyond Jesse's irascible, closed, and bitter exterior. When she told him about Reiki, Jessi reacted in a rude and pejorative manner. But when a wave of sharp pain stabbed his back, he quickly agreed to her trying to "demonstrate" some of the advantages of the method she had told him about. After a number of treatments, Jesse felt significant relief. No other treatment he had tried had helped so considerably. He had no choice but to admit that what she had said was true. After several treatments, the practitioner explained that he could use the method to treat himself, without being dependent on another practitioner. Every time he felt pain, he could alleviate it himself, without medication, and without other people.

These things touched Jesse's heart. He felt a fierce desire to learn the method himself, so that he could treat himself and would not have to be dependent on others, as he had been for such a long time, because of the accident. The idea that he could treat himself, and could bring relief and help to himself, seemed marvelous to him, even though he found it a bit hard to believe. However, the results were so blatant that he decided to try and learn Reiki in order to administer self-treatment.

After doing the first degree in Reiki, Jesse began to treat himself. The relief he felt was not only physical.

The mental changes that he underwent were very significant. He felt that suddenly his thinking had become more flexible, more open to listening, understanding, accepting things that in the past he would have rejected in an instant. He related to people in a gentler and more understanding way, and suddenly his life seemed less black, sad, and difficult. When he began to treat other people, Jesse was already a different person in his perception of the world. He did the second degree in Reiki, continued administering treatment, and saw wonderful results. By means of Reiki, Jesse's "weakness," the huge suffering he had known, the pain and the injuries, became the source of his strength and power. From them, he was able to make contact with people, and to understand them and be empathetic with their pain and feelings. He quickly became a successful and sought-after practitioner, and went on to become a Reiki Master.

When Jesse told me his story while we were sitting in the large institute for the study of Reiki and other healing methods that he managed, it was difficult for me to believe that the self-confident, smiling, serene, and charismatic man opposite me had been a bitter, irritable, hurt person, who felt anger and resentment toward the whole world. He went on to say that today he thinks about how he could have gone on living with the severe pains, but he could not have gone on living "life" in the true sense of the word with his negative and pessimist attitude. His life is now full of satisfaction and happiness, and the optimistic, compassionate, hopeful, and grateful view of life that he embraced enables him to enjoy every new and fascinating day, and remain steadfast in the face of life's vicissitudes.

*

Having said this, there is one pitfall of which the aware person, learning to treat himself as a way of increasing his personal awareness and his mental and spiritual growth, must beware.

Many methods of self-awareness and self-treatment are occasionally liable to turn into a way of shirking the basic problems that are inherent in a person's life. When a person suffers from a significant lack of balance in his life, or goes through a severe mental and physical crisis, he has to know that the methods of self-treatment, among them Reiki, do not constitute, in most cases, a substitute for professional help. This is true for an acute mental condition, as well as for a poor physical condition, chronic disease, and so on. The person must be aware and honest with himself, and know when to reach out for help. When one's troubles seem too overwhelming and difficult to deal with, at that moment, it is important to go and seek professional help. The suitable medical, psychological and holistic treatment, in combination with daily Reiki treatment, full body treatment and self-treatment, will constitute a successful whole with greater chances of achieving optimal balance and health.

In the same way, it is important for the person to understand that even if he administers self-treatments of Reiki on a daily basis, but does not make far-reaching, conscious, and serious changes in his way of life, thinking, and beliefs, if he continues with a way of life that is detrimental to him and the environment, the Reiki treatment will be no more than a "symptomatic" treatment. This is also the case when the person wants to improve his physical condition by means of self-treatment with Reiki, but does not pay sufficient attention to the other aspects of physical-mental health: correct nutrition, exercise, abstaining from harmful habits, and so on. A person who treats himself with Reiki, but eats unhealthily, for instance, or obstinately continues to adhere to unwanted characteristics, such as nervousness, sadness, anger, intolerance, and so on, will find that Reiki is ultimately of very little assistance to him.

Despite Reiki's tremendous power, and its physical, mental, and spiritual influence, the treatment itself is not enough. The person must make a conscious effort to go deeply into himself, to examine his way of life and his behavior, and try, in a clear and conscious way, to repair what needs fixing, those patterns of thought, belief, and behavior that limit and inhibit him. Many times, when we meet people who treat themselves, and maybe even others, with Reiki, and we observe their situation and way of life from the side, we feel that in fact, they have missed something, most likely because they did not undergo the deep and conscious change that is required in order to achieve spiritual and mental development, and true, lasting physical health.

Self-Treatment Procedure

This treatment takes 30-60 minutes, allowing the hand to remain on each of the following points for 3-5 minutes, but it is important to be aware of feelings and to operate according to intuition; that is, in a place that requires more Reiki, the hand should remain for a longer time. This treatment can be administered when you are sitting up, but you will probably be more comfortable lying down.

The Reiki points on the front of your body:

(When lying down, lie on your back.)

* Place each of your palms gently (without pressing) on each of your eyes. Remember that your arms must not be crossed, so that the correct way of placing your hands is right hand on right eye and left hand on left eye.
* Place each hand gently on each ear - right hand on right ear, left hand on left ear.
* Place both hands, one beneath the other, on the back part of the head.
* Place both hands on the throat, one on the other, or, if it more comfortable, your right hand on the right side of your neck, and your left hand on the left side of the neck.
* Place both hands on your chest. There are two ways of placing them; use one of them. It is possible to place one hand horizontally in the center of the chest, while the other hand is placed vertically below it in the center of the chest (on the sternum), so that a kind of cross is formed. The second possibility is to place one hand on each breast, gently, the right hand on the right breast, and the left hand on the left breast.
* Place your right hand on the right side of your solar plexus, which is located in the middle part of your chest (below the diaphragm), and your left hand on the left side of your solar plexus.
* Place your right hand on the right side of your waist, in line with your navel, and your left hand on the left side of your waist.
* Place both hands on the groin, in the form of a V.

The Reiki points on the back of your body:

(When lying down, lie on your stomach. Some people feel more comfortable treating the back of their body in a sitting position.)

* Place a hand on each shoulder. If you cannot place your right hand on your right shoulder and your left hand on your left shoulder (a certain degree of flexibility is required for this, and it is important that the treatment be relaxed and comfortable, without effort), there is no choice but to cross the hands, that is, place your left hand on your right shoulder, and your right hand on your left shoulder. In your thoughts, it should be clear that the crossing does not disrupt the flow of energy, and the energy flows directly and lightly with no interruption.

* Place a hand on each side of your waist, on your back, as high as possible.

* Place a hand on each side of your waist, behind your body.

* Place your right hand on your right buttock, and your left hand on your left buttock.

* This placement does not appear in some of the self-treatment books, but it is highly recommended: Place your right hand on your right knee, and your left hand on your left knee.

* Place one hand above your left foot, and your other hand below your left foot.

* Place one hand above your right foot, and your other hand below your right foot.

In addition, it is important to administer Reiki to every region in the body where there is a health problem, pain, or discomfort of any kind. Moreover, if you feel an intuitive need to place your hand on another region, even without a conscious reason, it is important to respond to this need and to administer a few minutes of Reiki to the region. While preparing to treat the mental level, it is possible to place your hands on regions of the body that are linked to various emotional phenomena: on your liver, in order to release angers; on your kidneys, in order to release guilt feelings; on your knees, in order to treat obstinacy and the inability to accept anything new; on your genitals, in order to cope with problems of accepting femininity/masculinity or various sexual problems (frigidity, impotence, insufficient pleasure during sexual intercourse, and so on).

The Degrees of Reiki

As we mentioned before, Reiki is not a regular holistic "profession" that can be studied in a regular manner - sitting in a classroom with a notebook, listening to lectures given by a teacher. It's not like that. Reiki's uniqueness lies in the fact that it is transmitted personally from teacher to pupil, and after the transmission of Reiki - the "attunement" - the pupil has the ability for the rest of his life. Of course, it would be good if he used it. The ability to be Reiki's life energy channel, and the ability to transmit it via the palms, can be used both for self-treatment and for treating others. When the Master transmits the healing ability to the pupil, he sketches extremely powerful sacred signs in the air in front of the pupil, and at his side. Some people have described their feeling at that moment, with their eyes shut, as a ticklish sensation in their palms, of energy flowing in their palms, of white light descending from above and passing through the crown of their head until it fills their entire body, and many other sensations. Other people do not feel any sensation, and even so, the energy still filters in and reaches them.

Reiki has a number of stages or degrees. First of all, the pupil achieves the first degree, that is attunement to the first degree of Reiki. In the attunement to the first degree, the Master teaches the pupil the history of Reiki, and sometimes various meditations are performed, preparing the pupil for Reiki attunement. During Reiki attunement, the Master uses his symbols to stimulate the pupil's energy centers and the chakras in the palms, by means of which he will administer treatment later on.

After attunement, the pupil learns to administer treatment by placing his hands on certain spots on his own body, and on that of the recipient.

A Full Treatment, Reiki First Degree

After the attunement to Reiki, the pupil is already allowed to administer treatment. As we mentioned before, a full treatment begins at the top, that is from the head, downward, toward the feet. In a full treatment, it is really a good idea if the recipient lies comfortably.

Reiki treatment is done with both practitioner and recipient fully dressed. It is very important to ensure that the hands do not rest directly on a woman's breasts, or on the groin of either sex, in order to prevent unpleasantness; they should be held a couple of inches above those regions. If the recipient feels uncomfortable when hands are placed on his eyes, the hands should be held a couple of inches above his eyes. In any event, care must be taken not to block his nostrils by mistake. Moreover, placing the hand on the throat is liable to be unpleasant for many people, so it is a good idea to hold the hand a couple of inches above the throat. Similarly, if a recipient shies away from contact, the treatment should be administered holding the hands a couple of inches above his body, without touching it.

We start the treatment from the head. There are a few procedures for placing the hands, and experienced practitioners sometimes add a couple of extra points to the treatment, according to the needs of the recipient.

The known procedure begins with linking up, that is, requesting assistance from the Reiki helpers. It is also possible to imagine the picture of one of the great Reiki Masters, or the Master who attuned the practitioner, while requesting assistance. We place our palms close to each other, in a gesture of prayer or beseeching, which is both customary and effective. After linking up and performing protections (to be discussed), we can begin the treatment.

* We ask the recipient to lie down on his back, and inform him that later on we will ask him to turn over onto his stomach.

* We stand behind or at the side of the recipient's head, and place our palms on his eyes. We leave our hands there for between three and five minutes, but in principle, an alert and experienced practitioner will listen to the energy flow. When the recipient needs energy in a particular region, it is possible that the practitioner will feel a sensation of some kind of suction or warmth in his palms, and so on. Sometimes, when the recipient has received as much energy as he can take at this stage, he will feel a kind of sensation of "rejecting" the energy, or a need to move the practitioner's hands off the spot.

Placing hands can be performed while glancing at a clock, but the best way is simply to pay attention to the inner feelings, and identify whether the placing of hands on that particular region should continue, and when to remove them.

* The ears: Laying of hands on the recipient's ears does not appear in the basic procedure according to Usui, but many practitioners are in the habit of relating to this spot. The hands should also be placed on the ears for three to five minutes, but again, you should heed your inner feeling, and act accordingly.

* The temples: This is the second point according to Usui's procedure.

* Behind the head: Place both hands, in a cupped position, below the recipient's head.

* The clavicle: Placing the hands on this region is related to the organs of the chest cavity. Place your hands comfortably on either side of the clavicle. Some place their hands on the throat before treating this point.

* Lower ribs: Placing the hands on the lower ribs when in fact part of the palm is placed on the region below the ribs, also relates to the kidneys and the organs in the lower abdomen.

Now there are three additional points that are used by many practitioners, but are not found in Usui's basic procedure:

* Above the groin: Hands are not placed directly on the groin, but rather just above it. This point is very important and significant, and the practitioner will often feel a very strong need to transmit energy to this region, so it should not be omitted.

* On the knees: This is a superb point for softening obstinacy and the reluctance to change patterns of life, thought, and belief. There are many people who need

treatment in this area, of course, beside the physical treatment of the knee joints, which in many people are places that are inclined to be injured, worn out, or easily hurt.

* On the feet: On the top of the feet, or on the sole, according to the practitioner's feeling.

Now ask the recipient gently and quietly to turn over and lie on his stomach.

*Shoulders: Place your hands on the recipient's shoulders, a place in which a heavy burden of tension, tasks, and responsibility accumulates. Let your hands remain there for as long as necessary, one hand on each shoulder, without crossing your hands.

* Lower back: Place your hands on the recipient's coccyx region.

Balancing the Chakras

Balancing the chakras is a treatment that has a great effect, both physically, and mentally and spiritually. Even after first-degree Reiki attunement, it is possible to administer treatment for balancing the chakras. After learning the symbols, you should use the appropriate ones in order to achieve more profound results. Although the results of the treatment will vary from person to person, the focus will be on the areas in which there is a problematic feeling, pain, or some kind of discomfort. Moreover, in the treatment we will try to work on the endocrine glands. Mrs. Takata prepared a basic treatment procedure that covers all the endocrine glands, whose importance for the general harmony of the body is crucial. The endocrine glands, which are activated by glands that are located in the brain, are directly responsible, from the physical point of view, for the homeostatis (the basic balance) of the body, and by releasing the hormones, they exert a tremendous influence on the person's mood and emotional state. From the ethereal point of view, these glands are linked to the seven major chakras.

The chakras are energy centers in the human body. There are many energy centers in the human body, but most healers concentrate on balancing the seven central chakras, a process that leads to the general balancing of the person's body, soul, and spirit. The meaning of the word "chakra" is "wheel." Accordingly, each chakra is manifested in the physical body as one of the endocrine glands that regulate all the physical and mental processes in the human body. Higher energies, cosmic energies, are channeled to the physical human bodies via the chakras. This energy, which is also called "life energy" that flows through the chakras, is of cardinal importance to our lives and health - physical, mental, and spiritual. When a situation arises in which the energy does not flow through the chakras in a harmonious way, or when one of the chakras is blocked, or is too open, an imbalance is created which is manifested in every aspect of life.

An imbalance in the state of the chakra will also come to the fore in the endocrine gland that is linked to it, and the delicate metabolic balance of the body will be disrupted. In the physical body, the chakras function as "broadcasters." They broadcast the currents that arrive from the higher and more distilled energy, which operates on the higher frequencies of energetic bodies, to the physical body, while "converting" the frequency to one that our physical body can utilize. The body that absorbs and contains the person's "soul" is the spiritual conscious body, which is our divine side that links us to creation. From this link, the energy passes to the other conscious bodies, each of which has a different vocation and purpose, and therefore requires energy of a different quality and a different frequency. On each "surface" there are stations that convert the energy for the next surface. The whole universe is linked by a tremendous, ancient force. This force is transferred to every thing and every creature according to its capacity, and in accordance with the frequencies that are appropriate to it, from the physiological, emotional, intellectual, and spiritual point of view. When this energy makes its way from this tremendous, ancient force to the bodies that are found in the universe, its strength and power ostensibly keep on diminishing, so that those bodies can absorb it, because by nature they do not contain even a minuscule fraction of its power.

The human body, like the universe, consists of different layers - a spiritual layer, an emotional layer, an intellectual layer. The difference between the human body and the "body" of the cosmos resides only in the length of their waves and frequencies. For that reason, the divine power is found not only outside of us, but also within us. Since human beings are capable of using the gift of the imagination, they can direct themselves intellectually, intuitively, or emotionally toward the various energy bodies and layers of awareness, and change them. All the methods that broaden consciousness, such as positive thinking, guided imagination, meditation, and many others, do this.

Every chakra serves as a relay station and message for the particular area of frequency or awareness. When we treat one of the chakras with Reiki energy, we are able to balance it, thus helping to balance the activities for which that particular chakra is responsible. The changes that occur in the wake of balancing the chakras can manifest themselves consciously or unconsciously in the recipient's physical, emotional, or spiritual layer, according to his essential needs at that time. This ensures his continued development and spiritual growth, and also balances his emotional state and gets him into a state of better physical health.

Besides the endocrine glands, the chakras are also linked to particular colors, to various physical, mental, and spiritual functions. For this reason, balancing them exerts an amazing influence on all the bodily and mental functions, and on raising the level of awareness and spiritual openness. Before we describe how to use Reiki to balance the chakras, we will briefly describe the activities of each of the chakras.

The first chakra - the base chakra

This is also called the root chakra. It is located between the anus and the genitals. This chakra is linked to man's basic survival instinct, to his existential fears, to his ability to be practical and to function successfully in the material world, to his ability to have both feet planted firmly on the ground, and to make decisions. It links the spiritual ability to the physical expressions of this ability. An imbalance in this chakra manifests itself in anxiety, aggression, a lack of confidence, and detachment. From the physical point of view, this chakra is linked to the whole spinal column and skeleton, to the body's excretory organs, and when it is not balanced, there are skeletal and joint problems, constipation and hemorrhoids, and so on.

The colors of this chakra are black and red.

The second chakra - the sex chakra

This chakra is located on the pelvis, between the pubic bones. It symbolizes change and individuality, while understanding other people's uniqueness. It is linked to pleasure, sexuality, desire, and fertility, which are its emotional and spiritual expressions, besides its physical expression. Moreover, this chakra is responsible for creativity, for self-realization, and for devotion to one's personal path. When the chakra is not balanced, the results will be many unrequited passions that the person tries to fulfill in all kinds of ways (such as an addiction to sex or food, and so on), restlessness, and sexual imbalance. From the physical point of view, this chakra is also linked to the excretory organs, to the muscles of the body, and to the sexual organs. The color of this chakra is orange.

The third chakra - the solar plexus chakra

This chakra represents the ego, and it houses the source of all feelings and sensations, doing, power, self-will, the "I," and the realization of the "I." Via this chakra, the person links up with the outside world and interprets it according to the balance of the chakra. A lack of balance in this chakra is manifested in manipulativeness, an unbalanced ego, domination, and an abuse of power. From the physical point of view, this chakra is linked to the respiratory system and the diaphragm, to the stomach, the pancreas, the gall bladder, the small intestine, the adrenal glands, and the sympathetic nervous system. The color of this chakra is yellow.

The fourth chakra - the heart chakra

This chakra is located in the center of the chest, parallel to the heart. It links the upper chakras to the lower ones, and is linked with the ability to love, to give unconditionally, to receive love, to forgive, and to show compassion. When this chakra is blocked, the whole body is affected by the blockage. From the physical point of view, this chakra is linked to the heart, the circulatory system, the lungs, the immune system, the thymus gland, and the hands. The colors of this chakra are pink and green.

The fifth chakra - the throat chakra

This chakra is located in the throat. It is linked to the ability to communicate with one's surroundings, and to all aspects of communication. It is responsible for the person's ability to express himself, for creativity, for belief, and for self-image. It links thought and its expressions. When the chakra is blocked, there are communication problems, the inability to express thoughts and desires, a lack of creativity, and conflicts between emotion and logic. From the physical point of view, this chakra is linked to the throat, to the thyroid gland, to the nerves, to the ears, to the muscles, to the neck, and to the vocal cords. The color of this chakra is blue.

The sixth chakra - the third eye chakra

This chakra is located on the forehead, between the eyebrows. This chakra is the one that links the person to his subconscious, to the intuition, to the ability to understand cosmic insights and receive non-verbal messages. Moreover, it is responsible for the balance between the two hemispheres of the brain, the right and the left, that is, between intuition, emotion, and mysticism on the one hand, and rationality and logic on the other. It is also responsible for the person's ability to concentrate, for mental serenity, for wisdom, and for extra-sensory perception. When the chakra is blocked, there can be situations of depression, headaches, mental exhaustion, auditory and visual problems, and learning and comprehension problems. From the physical point of view, this chakra is linked to the brain and its organs, the eyes, the ears, and the nose. The colors of this chakra are purple and indigo.

The seventh chakra - the crown chakraThe seventh chakra - the crown chakra

The location of this chakra is in the center, or crown, of the head. This chakra is linked to higher awareness, to divine and cosmic insights, to the ability to link up to divine knowledge and universal light and love. An imbalance in this chakra is liable to manifest itself in a feeling of boredom and a lack of purpose in the person's life, and in an inability to open up to spiritual dimensions. The colors of this chakra are purple white, dazzling white, gold, and silver.

Sometimes, the imbalance is liable to appear first in one of the endocrine glands. Sometimes, it appears first in a certain function that is associated with one of the chakras. In any event, they affect and will affect each other, and a problem in either one of the systems - the chakra system or the endocrine system - will manifest itself in the other. Reiki has the ability to be absorbed in both systems simultaneously, while balancing both the chakras and the hormonal system.

It is very important to point out that all the chakras are of equal importance. Sometimes, people are inclined to focus on treating the upper chakras, because they are more "spiritual." But the chakras are influenced by one another, and there is no point trying to balance and focus on the upper chakras when the lower ones are not balanced! A problem in one of the chakras will affect all the others, so that we have to try to balance all of them simultaneously. When we place our hands, we can feel which areas are in greater need of energy, and we will leave our hands in those places for a longer time.

In order to balance the chakras, we use the following techniques:

* A full and complete Reiki treatment, as described in the chapter describing the full treatment.

* The standing technique - a shorter treatment, in which the practitioner stands beside the recipient, places one hand a few centimeters in front of the lower abdomen, and the other hand a few centimeters in front of the sacrum, that is, in front of the first chakra, the base chakra. The hand must be held above these places for two to three minutes, until the practitioner feels the flow of energy growing, and then weakening, showing that the chakras have received the requisite energy. In the same way, the practitioner continues to the next chakras:

the solar plexus chakra, which is located in the region of the diaphragm, and the heart chakra, in the chest region. The hands must also be held for a few minutes over those places, according to the feeling of the amount of energy they require. When the practitioner feels that he can move to the next chakras, he ascends and holds one hand over the throat chakra, and the second hand over the third eye chakra, in the region of the forehead, for a few minutes. Afterward, he places both hands above the recipient's head in order to balance the seventh chakra - the crown chakra. After a few minutes, the hands are lowered above the chakras until the first chakra is reached, directing the thought to the balancing and closing of all the centers. (After the treatment and opening the chakras so as to balance them, it is important to close them in order to conclude the treatment.)

When balancing the chakras, it must be remembered that every chakra has its own specific need for balancing from the point of view of the length of time the hands are placed, so it is a good idea to work intuitively, and let the hands remain in the place for as long as necessary. In addition, second-degree Reiki can also be used, together with symbols, for balancing the chakras.

Reiki Second Degree

After studying, practicing, and assimilating the first degree of Reiki, it is possible to receive the second degree, which includes the use of symbols. After the symbols have been bestowed, they will accompany the Reiki practitioner in every stage of treatment, both of himself and of others.

The second degree of Reiki, as well as the third, opens up a new range of possibilities to the Reiki practitioner. It could be said that the attunement for the second degree increases the "capacity" of the person who earns it. In the same way, his ability to transmit the healing energy, to cleanse energetically, and to assist in the healing process of the recipient and, of course, of himself, increases. In addition, this ability is likely to accelerate the treatment, and shorten its duration, while its effectiveness increases.

Another point that enriches the treatment substantially is the reinforcement of the ability to produce harmony between the mental and the emotional layers. With second-degree Reiki treatment, it is possible to reach the depths of the subconscious more easily, thus influencing patterns of thought, belief, and behavior, some of which are not conscious at all. This way of working helps in the treatment of various addictions, fears, and phobias, in inhibiting situations whose cause the person cannot understand, chains of similar negative events that seem to "hound" the person, while in fact their cause is buried in the depths of his consciousness, without him understanding that he is in fact responsible for them. Of course, that leads us to the karmic links, which are also treated with second- and third-degree Reiki. As a result of these wonderful abilities, it is possible to discern the personal development of awareness both in the recipients and in the practitioners themselves.

Another ability used by practitioners of second- and third-degree Reiki is the ability to transmit energy to various objects - "programming" objects. This is mainly effective concerning crystals and healing stones. It is possible to transmit the Reiki energy to crystals that can subsequently be transferred to a person who needs them. The transmission of Reiki via crystals considerably strengthens the healing power of the crystal, and adapts it to the specific needs of the person who needs it.

This is the place to point out one of Reiki's most unique properties: Reiki reaches the place that most needs it, and treats the most pressing problem. In order to clarify this point, we will give a simple example. A person comes for treatment with Reiki for back and neck pains. After the first treatment, or even the second and third, he does not feel appreciable relief. However, his feeling of constant agitation gradually decreases, and he experiences a feeling of inner serenity during the day. He is much more relaxed, he sleeps better, but for the time being does not feel an improvement in his back and neck pains. There is an important and essential answer to the question, "Why didn't his pains disappear immediately after a few treatments?" Sometimes, the person reckons that the problem from which he is suffering is the one that requires massive treatment, while in fact his body and soul feel that there are more urgent problems - ones that may even be the indirect cause of the problem that he thinks is the major one. Reiki will first go through the basic problem - in this case, agitation and a lack of peace of mind. After balance is restored in the unbalanced mental situation, the body will free itself up to "request" the help of Reiki in treating the other problem - the back and neck pains.

We must remember that the problem we consider the first and most important is not always really the basic and most important problem that should be treated immediately. Fortunately, Reiki "knows" to get to exactly the place where it is needed the most, and so there will be an improvement in unbalanced and acute situations - whether they are mental, physical or spiritual, and only afterward will there be an improvement in the annoying external symptoms.

Another ability enjoyed by the practitioners of second- and third-degree Reiki is that of sending long-distance Reiki. This ability has many and varied forms and possibilities. It enables us to send healing Reiki energy to people who are far away from us - even to people we do not know personally, but we know of their problems and suffering. We can also send Reiki to places that have been struck by catastrophes such as an earthquake or some other natural disaster. We can send Reiki to the rain-forests, or to the earth, in order to help it purify itself of the pollution caused by man. Of course, when one person sends Reiki in this way, the amount of energy sent is small, even minuscule, but should not be ignored. On the other hand, when a group of people who have undergone second-degree Reiki attunement get together and send Reiki to the earth, to the rain-forests, to places that are beset by poverty or famine, to prisoners of war, and so on, their action is powerful and meaningful. The larger and more united the group, the more it operates in a coordinated and streamlined way, the stronger and more significant its energetic action will be.

Moreover, it is possible to use Reiki energy in order to cleanse energetically - rooms, people, various places. The level of radiation in certain places can be lowered by sending Reiki energy, but sometimes, for that, a number of people who have undergone second-degree Reiki attunement are needed to work together to purify the place of radiation.

Second-degree Reiki has powerful abilities. We will describe two more of them, more significant ones. One of them is the ability to send Reiki to a number of people simultaneously. As we see, at this level, the limitations of quantity, distance, and time decrease. The second one is transmitting Reiki to traumatic events that occurred in the past. By sending Reiki to them, it is possible to "break" behavior patterns that stem from those traumatic events.

Reiki Symbols

As we mentioned before, the use of symbols begins with second-degree Reiki. What are these symbols? Reiki symbols are the symbols that Dr. Usui received when he received the gift of Reiki. The symbols themselves contain the intentions of healing. With their help, it is possible to use additional powers that anyone who has not received second-degree Reiki attunement cannot use. Even if someone were to receive drawings of the symbols, there is no way he could use the power that they contain without second-degree Reiki attunement. These three symbols are the expression of Reiki's healing energy. The second-degree Reiki practitioner, and the Master - the third-degree Reiki practitioner - use them for self-healing, for healing others, and for sending long-distance Reiki. Working with symbols greatly reinforces the transmission of energy, as well as shortening the treatment time and increasing its power. Each symbol has a different meaning; they are used for different actions, separately and together, during a Reiki treatment, or sending long-distance Reiki using various techniques.

The Reiki symbols must be sketched in their correct form, and Reiki healers must remember them clearly, so that they can meditate with them easily, and see them in their mind's eye at any moment. It is highly recommended for them to try and draw each Reiki symbol about 10 times for 10-20 minutes each day, without looking at the page on which they are drawing, until they can sketch the sacred symbols perfectly. A mistake in outlining the symbol does not cause any damage, since Reiki is a universal energy of love, which only heals and does no harm. However, the incorrect outlining of the symbol is liable to undermine its effectiveness, or may not attain the desired result - if there is a result at all. It is therefore extremely important to persist in practicing and memorizing the symbols, until they become second nature, and flow naturally during treatment.

The first symbol - Cho Ku Rei

The first Reiki symbol is the symbol of power. It is spiral-shaped, and is used for bestowing strength and power, and for reinforcing the self-healing power of the body, soul, and spirit. It strengthens the power of Reiki, and is used to purify rooms, vehicles, and means of transportation in which non-positive energies can be felt, by transmitting a pure white light into these spaces. This symbol also serves as a protection, for charging the other symbols, for purifying food and drink, and for visualizing any part of the body - physical or mental.

The symbol can be outlined clockwise - that is how it relates to heaven, or the "masculine" energy, or anti-clockwise - that is how it relates to earth, or the "feminine" energy. When the two directions are combined, they can be used for charging other symbols, and for sketching the symbol of the Karia in the Krona Reiki method, which we will discuss later on.

The second symbol - Sei Hei Ki

The second symbol is the symbol of thought and feeling, and is extremely significant in the treatment of old, inhibiting patterns of belief, thought, and emotion. It means that God and man are one. It is superb for emotional and mental balance, and for creating balance between emotion and rationality, and between the two sides of the brain: the right brain, which is responsible for the actions of the left side of the body, and for creative and emotional activities, and the left brain, which is responsible for the actions of the right side of the body, and for logical, verbal, and analytical activities. Balance between the two parts of the brain leads to the attainment of a feeling of serenity, harmony, and inner peace. In principle, Reiki energy reaches every place that needs it. Therefore, when we want to treat the emotional body, we will avail ourselves of this symbol. The use of the symbol for attaining mental balance and treating old, unnecessary, and inhibiting thought patterns soon leads to the attainment of emotional balance and to far-reaching changes in the way of life. On this topic, it is important to point out that the reality that we experience is to a large extent the reflection of our beliefs and thought patterns - some of them conscious, and some unconscious. Many of them stem from childhood, from traumas that originated in events that were awful and traumatic in the eyes of a small child, but not so difficult and frightening in the eyes of an adult. As a result of the accumulation of these traumas, which were repressed in the subconscious, many adults exhibit irrational fears and illogical, inhibiting, and disruptive thought patterns.

Another type of thought and belief pattern comes from the things that were said to the child when he was young, as well as during his adolescence. Because of his unconditional faith in adults, he internalized these declarations as absolute truth. Statements such as "You're a loser," or declarations that were uttered among the adults, such as "All men are the same; they don't care about their wives..." and so on - severe and limiting declarations - become inhibiting patterns of thought and belief that the adult carries with him, without disagreeing with them or appealing them. In most cases, he is not truly conscious of the root of his inner beliefs. These beliefs will materialize in his life, and will become the reality of his life. The same child who was labeled a "loser" is liable, one way or another, to have this declaration come true in his adult life.

Many people are not aware of these inhibitions. They ask themselves why those same limiting scenarios, such as marital problems, a constant shortage of money, and so on and so forth, keep on occurring in their lives. Reiki treatment with this symbol may well raise these thought patterns to the conscious level. Sometimes, a change occurs in the person's thinking, without him even being conscious of it. Sometimes, he is struck by the knowledge that he has spent his life dragging inhibiting patterns like these behind him. Sometimes, he will recall experiences in which these thought patterns or various childhood memories were forced on him. It makes no difference how the inhibiting patterns of thought and belief are changed, but the minute it happens, the person is likely to experience far-reaching changes in his life; limitations that plagued him for years will suddenly be removed, and he will begin to feel, think, and believe in a different reality -

one that is better and more correct for his adult life. Very frequently, the change in patterns of thought and belief also changes or heals physical problems whose source lies in the direct or indirect after-effects of these thoughts or beliefs, which exert a significant influence on the processes in the body. Many psychosomatic illnesses such as asthma and so on are cured by treating inhibiting patterns of thought and belief.

Besides its use for mental and emotional treatment, the second symbol also serves to improve memory, learning, and understanding, to break bad habits such as smoking, overeating, and so on, to treat unbalanced emotions that disrupt everyday life, to remove negative energies from the chakras, to improve marriage and conjugal life, to soothe the conscious brain and achieve serenity and inner quiet, to cleanse the subconscious of traumas and residual baggage, to treat numerous problems of imbalance in children, and to alleviate emotional changes and confusion during adolescence. Another use - exceptional, perhaps, among the touch therapies - is in locating forgotten objects, events, people, names, telephone numbers, and so on.

The third symbol - Hon Hash Hez Venosh

The name of the third symbol means "The God within me blesses the God within you for bringing healing and enlightenment." This symbol is the most important of the symbols for long-distance Reiki treatment. Because it has no limitations of distance, time, or space, it can be used for changing past traumas (together with the second symbol, for instance), various karmic problems, and so on. It is used for sending Reiki to people and to past and present events, and for constructing a communication bridge between sender and recipient. It is used for sending Reiki anywhere in the world - to any person, object, event, or situation. It can be sent to future events or situations, such as an important meeting, an exam, and so on, in order for the Reiki energy to be present during the event, influence it in a beneficial way, and help accomplish the objective in a healthy, serene, and optimal manner. It is very effective when it is sent to a traumatic event in the past, which we want to erase from our present life, together with its influence, as well as to any unpleasant event whose memory and influence we want to erase. Of course, it can be used when we want to administer treatment without physical contact, because it strengthens this kind of treatment wonderfully, in a similar way to its influence on long-distance treatments. It can be used for treatment when we do not want to place our hands on the recipient's groin or breasts, when the recipient does not feel comfortable with physical contact for some reason, or is afraid of it, or when, because of a physical condition such as a burn or an infected or open wound, it is impossible or forbidden to place our hands on the recipient's body.

Reiki Third Degree, and the Master

The third degree of Reiki is the degree of Master. After receiving attunement for the third degree - the degree of Master - these people can help others become transmitters of Reiki themselves. The uniqueness of Reiki Masters, as opposed to other masters, lies in the fact that they are not part of any "superior organization." They are their own masters, and they are motivated by the desire to transmit Reiki in the world, and to help many other people by transmitting and teaching it.

At the level of Master, more symbols are added to Reiki treatment. Some of the symbols are not known to everyone; some of them were discovered and introduced into use by the revered Master, Bahagavan Sari Satia See Baba. The fourth symbol, Dai Ku Meo, is the symbol of the Master, and with its help, the Master administers treatment, and also gives attunement and training, so as to qualify new practitioners and initiate them in Reiki. Some people divide the third degree into Master and Master Teacher. The different methods have different divisions, but the form of the third degree that is accepted by most Masters is that of "Master and Master Teacher" simultaneously.

The fourth symbol - Dai Ku Meo

This is Usui's Master symbol. It operates at higher frequencies than the first symbol, Cho Ku Rei. When a more effective and speedy result is desired, or when there is a need for substantial or immediate healing, this symbol, in conjunction with the first symbol, Cho Ku Rei, has an astoundingly powerful action. When this symbol is used, it enables the energy and the unlimited divine wisdom to manifest themselves on the physical-material plane. It focuses and greatly reinforces the power of Reiki for attaining a stronger and speedier result, and leads to a greater feeling of perfection, unity, and fullness. Its use strengthens and blesses any action. Since it is a symbol with a karmic action and significance, many Masters recommend that it not be used for regular or general treatments, but only for attunement for Reiki by the Master, and for self-reinforcement by means of daily meditation.

The fifth symbol - Zonar

This symbol was introduced by Bahagavan Sari Satia See Baba. It is used in treating karmic problems, problems of previous lives, or problems in the present that are influenced by previous lives. It is very effective in treating various emotional problems. It is used for removing traumas from the subconscious, for treating problems that stem from karma or from previous lives, and for treating children and adults who were physically, mentally or sexually abused in childhood.

The sixth symbol - Harthi

This symbol, which is pyramid-shaped with a cross in its center, symbolizes love, truth, beauty, harmony, and balance. Like the fifth symbol, this symbol was introduced by Bahagavan Sari Satia See Baba. It is used for treating emotional problems and for any situation or problem concerning the heart - the center of love, receiving, and giving. It is also used in cases of unhealthy relationships, or problems in the relationships between family members, parents and children, siblings, couples, and close friends, and in treating any problem that might arise. It helps develop the krona - a Sanskrit word that means "an action full of compassion," which symbolizes a profound situation of "Love thy neighbor as thyself" - love and compassion for another person deriving from a feeling of unity and the understanding that we are all one; this implies that another person's pain and suffering are in fact our own pain and suffering. The symbol can be used in order to increase the will and lust for life, and for that reason it is good for use with seriously ill or terminal patients who have lost the will to live, with frail infants whose lives are in danger, and with anorexic people or people whose actions indicate that their natural will to live is defective (people who live in a way that leads to a slow death, a destructive and dangerous lifestyle, and so on). It can be used for rebuilding love and the desire for a normal career and profession, for treating addictions, and for meditation. People who used it during meditation report that it causes an extremely powerful and arousing experience.

The seventh symbol - Halu

This symbol was also introduced by Bahagavan Sari Satia See Baba, and it constitutes a kind of addition to and completion of the fifth symbol, the Zonar, enhancing its action; it is therefore stronger, and operates on higher levels. This symbol is used for deep healing and for restoring physical, mental, and spiritual balance, for treating mentally deficient children, for breaking negative mental patterns - even the deepest and strongest ones - for attaining higher awareness, and for treating cases of physical or sexual abuse, rape in the family, battered women, and so on. Moreover, it is used for releasing karma.

The eighth symbol - Rama

This symbol is used for linking up with the earth and the spirits of heaven. It is used for opening and balancing the lower chakras, for balancing the lower and upper chakras, for cleansing rooms of negative energies, for purifying crystals, for strengthening and reinforcing objectives and the ability to accomplish them. (Of course, it should be used for clean and pure objectives for the benefit of humanity in general. It is not at all desirable, to put it mildly, to use it for objectives that are not pure, or that are unhealthily selfish.) Moreover, the symbol is also used for various grounding purposes as well as protection, such as the protection and grounding of vehicles, plants, and so on, against accidents, and safeguarding property and money in businesses.

The ninth symbol - Gnossa

The ninth symbol is used for joining the person more closely to his "upper I," and for receiving higher awareness and bringing it to the physical body, while creating suitable awareness. It is used before meditation connected to the crown chakra in order to created a connection with the "upper I," and in order to reinforce the force of a crystal web and its charging.

The tenth symbol - Eah Vah

This symbol creates our reality as our exclusive reality, without anyone else's influence or radiation. It is used for radiation onto plants that are in danger of wilting in order to revive them, for turning missions and projects that are still at the conceptual stage into realities in the physical world, and for realizing aims and ambitions.

The eleventh symbol - Shanti

The eleventh symbol releases fears and anxieties, nightmares and bad dreams, and affords a harmonious and peaceful life in the present. In this way, it helps create a better, more peaceful, and more harmonious reality. It is used in conjunction with the tenth symbol, Eah Vah, for expressing ambitions and desires in the physical world, for their physical realization, for healing the past, for opening the third eye, and for cleansing and completing the aura, while reaching a state of calm, peace, and serenity.

In addition to these eleven symbols, there are many additional symbols, which certain Masters transmit to their pupils during attunement and by studying, such as the symbol of the Dragon's Fire, as well as the symbols of gratitude, peace, Jupiter, Lan-Su-Mei, Midas Star, Trinity, and many others. Most of them can be charged with the first Reiki symbol, Cho Ku Rei, so as to enhance their activity. But it is extremely important to remember that Reiki symbols have their own meaning, and, one could say, their own "personality." For this reason, they must be used for the correct purposes, and with total respect. That is, they must not be used too "liberally" or casually, but the right symbol at the right place and time, for the appropriate use. Daily meditation with one of the symbols with which you feel comfortable meditating - a symbol whose meaning is necessary for you to enhance your power to heal and benefit, and for your spiritual development - is very powerful and arousing, and contains multiple experiences. In accordance with the principle of gratitude, one of Reiki's five principles, and out of respect and thanks, it is important to thank every symbol before and after using it. Moreover, this gratitude will reinforce the power of the symbol and will make it more effective and powerful when it is used.

Krona Reiki

After learning many principles and methods of treatment according to "Usui Reiki," it is worthwhile taking a look at one of the most accepted methods of Reiki, "Krona Reiki."

Krona is a Sanskrit word, used in turn in Hinduism, Buddhism, and Zen, meaning "action full of compassion." This compassion means that when a person is enlightened, he sees no difference between people, and his compassion-filled action reaches every person, without discrimination or differentiation, since he sees all human beings as one whole, including himself. According to this perception, the very fact of the tremendous desire to relieve the suffering of others, who are not really perceived as "others," but rather as part of the whole, creates two situations. First, the desire and enlightened perception strengthen the desire itself and turn it into a realistic action. The second is by seeing all human beings as one, by a perception of unity, the alleviation of the suffering of one man heals and helps the whole world. It is not an empty metaphor, but an energetic way of relating to the unity of our souls, which are influenced by one another limitlessly.

Krona Reiki has its own abilities, and it is no less powerful and significant than Usui Reiki. Krona Reiki operates simultaneously on the energy bodies, and its practitioners claim that it is more tangible and concrete. Moreover, they say that the energy of Krona Reiki surrounds them, and the recipients feel an additional sensation beyond the feeling of the energy that envelops them - that of beneficial grounding.

People who undergo Krona Reiki attunement experience a connection with their instructors, with their angels, and with their "upper I," as well as the healing presence of beneficent beings.

Similar to the marvelous work of Dr. Usui, who received Reiki and the special information through meditation and spiritual work, so too William Rand, the person who developed Krona Reiki, reached his realizations and enlightenment through meditation with Reiki symbols. By means of this meditation, he discovered ways of augmenting the power of the symbols, and of increasing their abilities. By means of this meditation, he himself went through attunement for Krona Reiki, and founded the new order.

Krona, that is, action full of compassion, is the quality of all the light beings that operate around us. They operate regularly, and their blessed light influences every creature. However, not every person has the ability to receive this light. What determines its final and healing influence is each person's individual ability to receive. The people who underwent attunement or training for Krona Reiki increase their ability to receive those blessed lights enormously, that is if they use them in order to help and benefit themselves and others, when, of course, according to this perception, they are all one. The uniqueness of this method, therefore, is that by working with it, it exposes us to closer work with the enlightened beings. We may encounter these beings in their ethereal or spiritual form, or possibly in human form, if it is necessary to work closely with them. People who are experienced in this type of Reiki relate wonderful things about the feelings that arise while receiving Reiki, and about the amazing results of treatment. However, the best result will be achieved from a merging of Usui Reiki and Krona Reiki. In any event, in order to send long-distance Reiki, the two methods should be combined.

Astrolog Publishing House

P. O. Box 1123, Hod Hasharon 45111, Israel

Tel: 972-9-7412044

Fax: 972-9-7442714

E-Mail: info@astrolog.co.il

Astrolog Web Site: www.astrolog.co.il

ISBN 965-494-102-3

Published by Astrolog Publishing House 2000

Printed in Israel

2 4 6 8 10 9 7 5 3 1